RESISTANCE BAND EXERCISE SIMPLIFIED

A COMPLETE GUIDE RESISTANCE BAND WORKOUT

JESSE SMITH

Table of Contents

CHAPTER ONE

Exercising with a resistance band

You can exercise your entire body with resistance bands, which are large elastic bands. Many of the exercises can be performed while seated, making them suitable for those with limited mobility.

We should all engage in muscle-strengthening exercises at least twice a week, according to BHF physical activity specialist Lisa Purcell.

Flexibility exercises help you perform everyday tasks more easily by increasing the range of motion in your muscles. They can all be done while sitting.

Your doctor or cardiac rehabilitation team should be consulted before embarking on any exercise program if you have a heart condition or high blood pressure.

Join the band and have some fun! Strength training and rehabilitation can benefit from the use of resistance bands. Size, length, and resistance levels are all available.

They're also easy to transport and store, making them ideal for home workouts, hotel workouts, or making the most of a limited gym space.

Exercise bands, like free weights, come in a variety of resistance levels, ranging from extremely stretchable to extremely strong.

Tubular band with handles and loop band are the most commonly used types of band. As a last resort, you can consult a fitness professional to help you choose the right band based on your current fitness level and workout plan.

Aim for 2 to 3 sets of 8-25 repetitions per exercise for the majority of your workouts. There's no time like the present!

Exercises for the lower body

Leg day is a must...

1. Squats in the front position

These are going to be great for your buttocks, thighs, and hamstrings! (after they stop burning). The groin, hip flexors, and calves can all benefit from front squats as well as the rest of your body.

It's how to get it done.

1.

You should place your feet slightly wider apart than shoulder-width apart on the band while standing on it.

2.

In each hand, hold a handle that extends the length of the band. If the band is too long, cross your arms at your chest to keep it in place.

3.

Relax as if you're taking a seat. Keep your chest up, your abs firm, and your feet flat.

4.

Return to your starting position.

5.

Count to 8–12 repetitions.

2. Extending one's leg

With this quad builder, you can take things up a notch.

Shar

It's how to get it done.

1.

Using a loop band, secure one end of the band to a support (like an incline bench) while the other end is looped around your ankle.

2.

Step away from the anchor and place your feet hip-width apart to create tension in the band.

3.

Right leg lifted from the floor, shift the weight to the left foot.

4.

Straighten your knee in front of you by extending it all the way out in front of you.

5.

Retrace your steps back to the starting point.

6.

Before switching legs, perform 8–12 reps of this exercise.

3. Leg curl in the prone position

Your hamstrings will thank you.

It's how to get it done

CHAPTER TWO

1.

Loop a band around your right ankle and secure it to a stable object close to the ground for support while lying face down.

2.

Create tension by moving away from the anchor.

3.

As far as you're able, bring your heel toward your glutes while tightening your core.

4.

Slowly bring your leg back to where it was before you began.

5.

Switch sides after 10–15 repetitions.

4. Bridge of glutes

Your glutes deserve a high five!

It's how to get it done.

1.

Loop a band around your right ankle and secure it to a stable object close to the ground for support while lying face down.

2.

Create tension by moving away from the anchor.

3.

As far as you're able, bring your heel toward your glutes while tightening your core.

4.

Slowly bring your leg back to where it was before you began.

5.

Switch sides after 10–15 repetitions.

4. Bridge of glutes

Your glutes deserve a high five!

It's how to get it done.

1.

Loop a band around your right ankle and secure it to a stable object close to the ground for support while lying face down.

2.

Create tension by moving away from the anchor.

3.

As far as you're able, bring your heel toward your glutes while tightening your core.

4.

Slowly bring your leg back to where it was before you began.

5.

Switch sides after 10–15 repetitions.

4. Bridge of glutes

Your glutes deserve a high five!

It's how to get it done.

1.

Tie a band around your thighs, just above the knees, and hold it in place.

2.

Place your hands on your hips and knees bent at a 90-degree angle.

3.

Raise your hips until your shoulders, hips, and knees are aligned by contracting your glutes and applying gentle pressure outward against the band.

4.

Do 15–20 repetitions.

5. Taking a step backwards

The adductor exercise is king when it comes to sculpting your hips, groin, and inner thigh.

It's how to get it done.

1.

Stand with your right side facing the support and wrap your free end around your right (outer) ankle after anchoring a loop band at ankle height to a support.

2.

Step away from the support and stand perpendicular to the band to create tension.

3.

Perform a quarter squat starting from a wide stance.

4.

Work against the resistance by pulling in your right leg toward your left.

5.

Retrace your steps back to the starting point. Before switching sides, perform 12–15 repetitions.

6. Clamshell

If you want to dance to Lizzo & Missy Elliott's song, you'll need to loosen up your external hip rotators and improve your range of motion and flexibility.

It's how to get it done.

1.

Just above the knees, tie an elastic band around yourself.

2.

Lie on your side with your knees and hips flexed to a 90-degree angle to begin.

3.

Pull your knees apart while contracting your glutes for 2–3

seconds while keeping your feet together.

4.

Retrace your steps back to the starting point.

5.

Perform 10–12 reps of each exercise.

7. Inversion of the foot

Even if it's not at the top of your priority list, keeping your ankles flexible will help you avoid more serious problems in the future.

This is even better news: You can take a break.

It's how to get it done.

1.

Lean forward with one leg straight and the other bent, and sit down.

CHAPTER THREE

2.

Wrap the middle of a resistance band around the ball of your foot while holding both ends.

3.

Straighten your back and point your toes away from you while sitting.

4.

Bring your toes back up and flex them toward your knee as far as you feel comfortable doing so in a controlled movement.

5.

Retrace your steps back to the starting point.

6.

Performing 10–12 reps on each side

8. Band walk in the lateral direction

Don't try to get around these obstacles!

It's how to get it done.

1.

Wrap a therapy or loop band around your lower legs, just above your ankles.

2.

To make the band tighter, stand with your feet shoulder-width apart.

3.

Take a half-squat as a starting point.

4.

Then, with your right leg, step sideways to your left, shifting your weight over to your left side. Keep the band taut, but move your standing leg slightly inward.

5.

Before going the other way, take 8–10 steps backwards.

9. On the spot kidnapping

It's a bit of a juggling act, this one. The glutes will thank you.

It's how to get it done.

1.

Wrap a band around your ankles and secure it with a knot.

2.

Step out to the side slowly while lifting your working leg. To activate your glutes, keep your foot pointed forward and lead with your heel.

3.

If you're feeling shaky, grab a strap or something similar for support (like the wall or the back of a chair).

4.

Make your way back to the starting point.

5.

Repeat on each side for 15–20 repetitions.

10. The kidnapping of a person while they are seated

Try a seated abduction to show your thighs who's in charge. As a result, you can sit back and relax.

.

It's how to get it done.

1.

To do this, you'll need to find a comfortable place to sit and a loop band to go around both of your knees.

2.

Take a few steps back and widen your feet.

3.

Keeping your feet firmly planted as you slowly widen your legs, slowly press your knees out.

4.

Bring your knees back to each other and hold for two seconds.

5.

Do 15–20 reps.

Arm strengthening exercises

Start a war of attrition.

11. The curl of concentration

Prepare for the upcoming gun show with these helpful hints. Your biceps will thank you.

CHAPTER FOUR

It's how to get it done.

1.

Place the middle of the band under your right foot while in a forward lunge position with your right leg in front of you.

2.

Place your elbow on the inside of your knee and hold the loop band in your right hand.

3.

Curl the band toward your shoulder while squeezing your biceps with your palm facing away from your knee.

4.

Slowly bring the band back to its original position.

5.

After 8–10 reps, switch sides and repeat.

12. Curl your biceps while standing.

If you're looking to build muscle in your upper body, this is a great way to do it. Crazy.

It's how to get it done.

1.

Standing over the middle of the band, your feet should be placed shoulder-width apart.

2.

Starting with your arms down at your sides, grab a handle with each hand.

3.

Bend your elbows and pull your arms toward your shoulders while keeping your palms facing forward until you feel a strong contraction in your biceps.

4.

Slowly return to the floor.

5.

Do 12 to 15 curls.

13. Reverse kickback with your quads

Relax and enjoy yourself. Joking aside, I'm not offended!

Tell others about it!

It's how to get it done.

1.

Lie on your back with your knees bent over the center of the band and your feet together.

2.

Position your arms at your sides, palms facing behind you, and hold the ends of the band.

3.

Bend your elbows so that your forearms are parallel to the floor, keeping them tucked in by your sides.

4.

After that, extend your arms as far as they will go by pressing down on them and pulling the band behind your back.

5.

Retract your steps.

6.

Work your way up to 8–10 repetitions.

14. Extend the triceps up overhead in this exercise.

For the sake of your biceps, become a triceps-ratops.

Share

It's how to get it done.

1.

Place a tube band around your glutes while sitting on a chair or bench.

2.

Stretch your arms up and bend your elbows so that your hands are behind your neck while holding a handle in each hand.

3.

Extend your arms to their fullest potential while keeping your palms facing the ceiling and your arms straight.

4.

Retract your steps.

5.

Switch sides and perform 10–12 reps on each side.

Strength training for the middle and lower body

These intense workouts will get you right to the heart of the matter.

CHAPTER FIVE

15. Crunches while on your knees.

The top of a door can be a great place to work your core.

It's how to get it done.

1.

Kneel down facing away from the anchor and attach the band to a high anchor (such as the top of a door or a cable column). Then, grab the band on either side and pull it over your shoulder with your elbows bent.

2.

Engage your core and crunch down toward your hips while contracting your abs by extending your elbows out at shoulder level.

3.

Retrace your steps back to the starting point.

4.

Ten to twelve repetitions should be completed.

16. Woodchopper

Get your biceps working hard.

It's how to get it done.

1.

To prevent it from slipping, place the loop or tube band at the very top of the strut.

2.

Grab the free end of the band with your arms extended overhead while keeping your right side toward the support.

3.

Pull the band diagonally across your body to the front of your knees in one fluid motion while rotating your right hip and pivoting your left foot.

4.

Retrace your steps back to the starting point. Work your way up to 8–10 reps on each side, then switch sides.

17. Band members walked out in protest of rotation

Walk away when necessary. Slowly.

It's how to get it done.

1.

Using a cable column or other support, fasten a small loop or tube band just below your rib cage.

2.

Squat down and grip the free end of the band with your free hand.

3.

Holding the band with both hands straight out in front of your chest, step laterally until the band is too tense to go any further.

4.

Return to the starting position by moving slowly and carefully back toward the column.

5.

Repeat six to eight times on each side.

18. Crunch in reverse

It's time to flip it around and do it the other way around now! (Missy stays winning throughout this article).

It's how to get it done.

1.

Secure the band to a low-lying surface.

2.

Your knees should be bent 90 degrees as you lie faceup.

3.

Make a tight band around the tops of both feet by scooting back.

4.

Contraction of the abdominal muscles causes the lower body to curl toward the shoulders. To bring your knees closer to your chest, lift your hips off the ground.

5.

Retrace your steps back to the starting point.

6.

Perform 12–15 reps of this.

19. An ethnic twist

CHAPTER SIX

It's how to get it done.

1.

Put your feet in a comfortable position on the floor, and then wrap the band around them from the center out.

2.

In both hands, hold the two ends that are not attached to each other.

3.

Lean back at a 45-degree angle while keeping your knees slightly bent.

4.

Right-handed people can rotate the band by crossing their hands across their bodies and putting their hands on their hips to the left and right.

5.

Bring the band toward your right hip while maintaining neutrality in your middle and low back by contracting your oblique muscles.

6.

Get back to where you were before.

7.

Rotate left and right for 10–12 reps on each side, alternating directions each time.

Exercising the back

Put your words into action and begin toning.

20. the rowdy bunch

Put your best effort into it.

Post to Pinterest.

It's how to get it done.

1.

Lie on your back with your knees bent and your feet shoulder-width apart over the band.

2.

Keep your hips back as you take a slight knee bend and a hinge at the waist.

3.

Bend at the knees and grasp the handles of the band with your hands facing outward.

4.

Pull the band up toward your hips, squeezing your shoulder blades together, until your elbows form a 90-degree angle, and then release the band.

5.

For 10–12 reps, lower yourself and row back up.

21. In-row seating

Get comfortable, but not too comfortable. Place the center of the band behind the soles of your feet while keeping your legs extended.

It's how to get it done.

1.

Take hold of the band with both hands, palms facing each other, as you spread your arms wide.

2.

Squeeze your shoulder blades together while bending at the elbows and bringing the band toward your core. If you find it easier to sit up straight if you bend your knees a little, do so.

3.

Retrace your steps back to the starting point.

4.

Perform 10–12 reps.

22. To dismantle

This should be a part of your workout if you want stable shoulders and better mobility.

It's how to get it done.

1.

Kneel slightly and place your feet shoulder-width apart as you stand.

2.

Using both hands, place them shoulder-width apart on the middle section of the band, palms facing down.

3.

The band should be pulled out and back until your shoulder blades begin to contract, keeping your arms straight.

CHAPTER SEVEN

4.

Retrace your steps back to the starting point.

5.

8–10 repetitions of stretching, squeezing, and releasing.

23. Pullover worn while lying in bed

Sadly, this does not entail hiding under the covers, but good try.

Post to Pinterest.

It's how to get it done.

1.

Anchor the tube band in a low position for this pec and lat exercise.

2.

Holding onto the free end of the band with both hands as you lie face down, extend your arms straight out in the air. Create some tension by moving away from the anchor.

3.

Pull the band overhead, crossing your torso until the handle reaches your knees, with your elbows slightly bent.

4.

Retrace your steps back to the starting point.

5.

Keep going for eight to ten repetitions.

24. Pulled down lats

You're ready to work on your upper back.

It's how to get it done.

1.

A horizontal bar should be used to secure the band in place (or even a sturdy tree limb).

2.

In order to keep the band in front of you, kneel with your back to the anchor.

3.

Extend your arms overhead and spread your hands slightly wider than shoulder width apart to hold each end tightly.

4.

Stretch out the band by bending your elbows and lowering it toward the floor while keeping your back muscles contracted.

5.

Slowly return your hands to the starting position after they have reached your shoulders.

6.

Do 10–12 rounds of this.

Exercises for the chest

Look no further for barrel pecs than here.

25. Push-up

Try out a new twist on a classic move.

It's how to get it done.

1.

Place the resistance band across your upper back as you hold a plank position.

2.

Start by placing your hands on the floor, palms facing the floor, with the ends of the band looped around your hands.

3.

Push yourself up until your arms are fully extended, contracting your glutes and abs.

4.

Your chest should be on the floor as you do this.

5.

For 5–20 repetitions, see what you can do (depending on your strength).

26. Chest press while inclined

Next, we'll focus on your biceps and pectorals!

It's how to get it done.

1.

To begin, sit down and wrap your band around an anchor in the back of your head.

2.

Bring the band to your shoulders, one handle in each hand.

3.

In order to fully extend your arms, press the bands upward straight above the chest.

4.

Retract your steps.

5.

Ten to twelve repetitions should be completed.

27. Pressing weights on a bench

What's this? There's no barbell? It's all good! When all else fails, reach for the resistance bands.

It's how to get it done.

1.

Then, with your feet flat on the bench, fasten a tube band around your wrists and head.

2.

Take a hold of a handle with each of your hands.

3.

Hands at shoulder height is a good starting point (so your thumbs touch the front of your shoulders).

4.

At the height of your reach, bring your hands together in front of your chest.

5.

Retract your steps.

6.

Ten to twelve repetitions should be completed.

The bench press and push-ups were put side by side to determine which exercise provided the best results in terms of building size in the chest. Find out by reading on.

28. Push-ups while standing

Getting a better chest is as easy as going to the beach.

CHAPTER EIGHT

It's how to get it done.

1.

Using a cable column or other sturdy support, secure the tube band at chest height.

2.

Do not turn your back on the band while grabbing each handle

3.

Position your hands at chest height as you step forward to reduce the slack.

4.

Press the band straight out in front of you until your arms are at their full extension, and then squeeze your chest muscles as hard as possible.

5.

Get back to where you were before.

6.

For a total of 12–15 repetitions, keep pressing.

Exercises for the Shoulders

Make yourself at home amongst the greatest minds of all time.

29. Overhead guillotine

You might not understand this one (in fact, it definitely should).

It's how to get it done.

1.

Stand with your feet shoulder-width apart over the center of a tube band.

2.

Grip each handle with your thumbs touching your shoulders and your palms straight forward.

3.

Extend your arms to their fullest extent by pressing straight up.

4.

Slowly retrace your steps.

5.

Work your way up to 8-10 repetitions.

30. Raising one's chin

Get to know this one because it's great for the front of your shoulders.

Tell others about it!

It's how to get it done.

1.

Hands facing back, thumbs pointing inward, stand shoulder-width apart on the middle of the band and apply pressure to the front of your shoulders.

2.

Bring your right arm straight out in front of you to shoulder height without locking your elbows.

3.

Slowly return to the floor.

4.

Before switching arms, perform 8–12 lifts on each arm.

31. Raising the lateral limbs

This isolation move will help you develop stronger shoulders.

Post to Pinterest.

It's how to get it done.

1.

Place your feet shoulder-width apart over the center of a tube band.

2.

As you grip each handle, keep your arms at your sides and your palms facing toward one another.

3.

Raises hands to shoulder height, slightly bending elbows at the wrists.

4.

Slowly return to the floor.

CHAPTER NINE

5.

Do 8–10 repetitions.

32. Rowing straight up and down

Be confident as you aim for your traps.

It's how to get it done.

1.

In order to get the most out of the band, place your feet shoulder-width apart over the

center of the band and grip the
handles with your palms facing
you.

2.

While keeping your elbows bent
and your body in a high V, pull
the band straight up your front
until it reaches your shoulders.

3.

Return to the starting position
by lowering your body slowly.

4.

Row for 10–12 repetitions.

If you prefer to row on a rowing machine, we've got some tips for you to follow.

33. Back delt fly with an unusual bend in it

Take aim at your entire shoulder with this powerful strike.

Tell others about it!

It's how to get it done.

1.

Stand with your feet centered over the band's center.

2.

Gripping both handles with your palms facing each other, you should be able to cross the band at your knees.

3.

Lift your arms straight out to your sides until the band reaches your shoulders, then bend forward at the waist with your back straight.

4.

Take a deep breath and lower yourself back to the beginning position.

5.

With 10–12 repetitions, take off.

Post to Pinterest.

Takeaway

At home, there's no need for a full-scale gym. Resistance bands, on the other hand, are a convenient and efficient way to

work every muscle group in your
body at the same time.

THE END